Fertility Diet CookBook

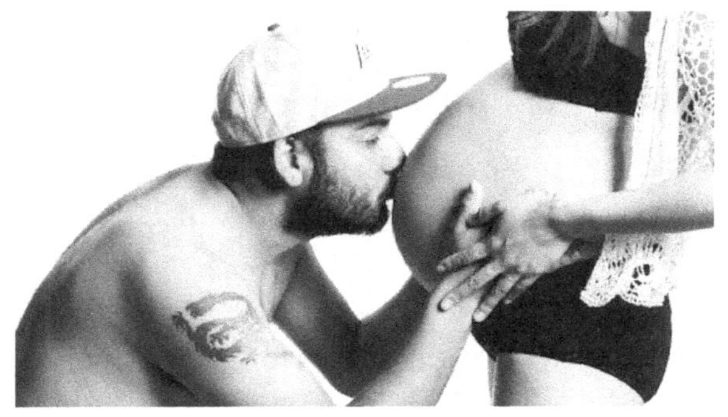

Quick and Easy Recipes to Boost Fertility in Women Over 35

Travis R. Burkhart

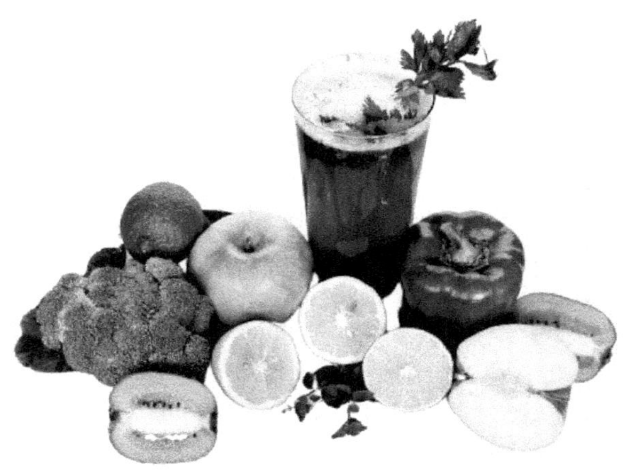

TABLE OF CONTENTS

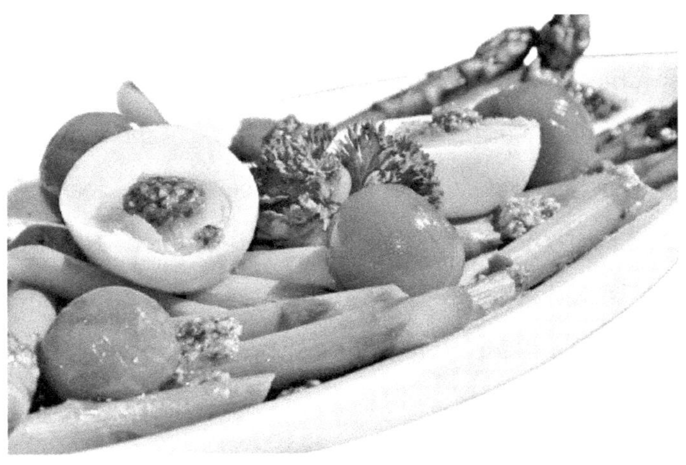

INTRODUCTION

A young woman named Elara used to reside in a charming village surrounded by lush meadows and rolling hills. Elara and her devoted husband Milo had always wanted a baby, but they were unable to conceive despite their undying love for one another.

Elara set out on a quest to learn the mysteries of fertility because she was determined to find a solution. She examined old manuscripts for solutions, conferred with healers, and asked knowledgeable elders for advice. Elara learned about the power of fertility foods—nutrient-dense meals said to improve reproductive health and aid in conception—through her quest.

Equipped with her newfound wisdom, Elara set out to grow an abundant garden full of foods that would increase fertility. She carefully and devotedly tended to rows of gorgeous fruits, aromatic herbs, and colorful veggies. Elara tended to her garden every day, giving the little seedlings words of encouragement as they sought the sun.

Elara's garden grew and produced an abundance of nutrient-dense, vibrant crops as the seasons changed. She carefully made healthy meals for Milo and herself, including a variety of foods high in nutrients that promote fertility in their daily diet. Together, they relished the tastes of sharp greens, fresh fruits, and robust grains, and with each satisfying mouthful, their sense of optimism was restored.

Elara felt a stirring of life within her, strengthened by the sweetness of nature's richness, a subtle reminder that miracles were possible even in the face of tragedy. She and Milo remained true to each other, welcoming the future with wide arms and unflinching faith.

And then, as the sun rose over the horizon one fateful morning, Elara heard the news that made her heart happy and wonderous. She was carrying the priceless gift of a new life within her, making her a dazzling light of promise and hope.

The locals marveled at Elara's garden's bounty and the love that grew among her family as her belly grew with the wonder of creation. They rejoiced at the birth of a long-awaited child, a monument to the strength of fertility foods and the resiliency of the human spirit, and toasted the wonder of life, recognizing the sacred tie between nature and nurture.

Thus, Elara and Milo welcomed their little wonder into the world in the center of the village, surrounded by fields of fragrant wildflowers and golden wheat. Their little miracle was formed from the seeds of life, fed by love, and destined to flourish forevermore among the beauty of their abundant garden.

Here at the Fertility Feast, each morsel you eat is a step closer to realizing your dream of becoming a parent. On this gastronomic adventure, we'll investigate how food may improve fertility, nourish your body, and reignite the spark of life within. Come along on a delectable journey towards the wonder of conception, filled with nutrient-rich foods and tasty meals made with love. So prepare to taste the sweetness of fertility as we uncover the techniques for nurturing your path to parenthood—grab your apron and sharpen your knives. Now let's get started!

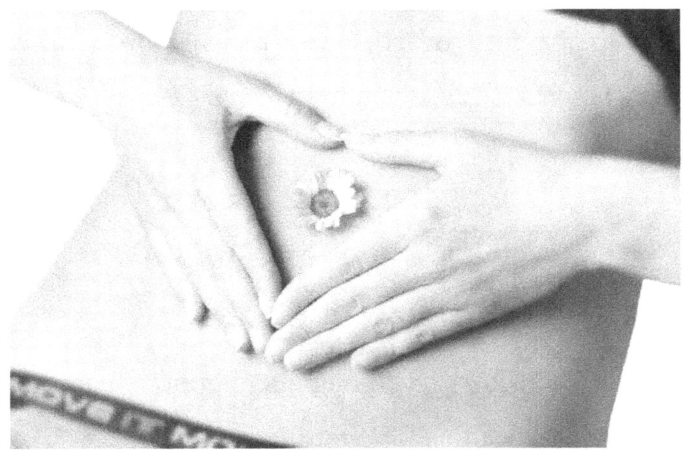

CHAPTER 1

Overview of Nutrition for Fertility

Welcome to the trip aimed at women over 35 to improve fertility with nutrition. In this chapter, we will examine the role that nutrition plays in maximizing reproductive health, discuss essential nutrients that are critical to fertility, and introduce you to the idea of preparing recipes for fertility. Let's go off on this adventure piece by piece.

Recognizing the Role Nutrition Plays in Fertility

Numerous factors, including age, hormone balance, and general health, affect fertility.

- Nutrition is essential for maintaining reproductive health since it influences menstrual cycle regularity, hormone production, and egg quality.

- Proper nutrition is even more important for women over 35 since they may experience particular issues connected to fertility due to age-related reductions in ovarian function and egg quality.

Examining Important Nutrients for Fertility

- Important nutrients that are essential for fertility are as follows:
- Folic acid: is necessary to protect the growing embryo from neural tube abnormalities.
- Iron: is essential for sustaining healthy blood hemoglobin levels and promoting the health of reproductive organs.
- Omega-3 fatty acids: These fats, which are present in walnuts, flaxseeds, and seafood, balance hormones and lessen inflammation.

- Antioxidants: These plant and nut-based compounds shield reproductive cells from oxidative harm.

- Together, these nutrients provide the best conditions for conception and pregnancy.

Outlining Fertility Recipe Preparation

- Cooking fertility recipes entails preparing foods high in nutrients that are proven to promote reproductive wellness.

- You can actively support your fertility journey by adding fertility-boosting components to scrumptious and nutritious recipes.

- To support general health and reproductive function, fertility recipe cooking emphasizes using whole foods, minimally processed components, and balanced meals.

Making Goals for Your Journey Toward Fertility

- Think for a moment about your aspirations and goals for fertility.
- Think about how diet can help you achieve these objectives and maintain the health of your reproductive system.
- Adopt a positive outlook and make a dedication to feeding your body with nutrients that support vigor and fertility.

Prepare to Take Off

- Assemble everything you'll need, including your preferred writing instrument and a notepad for recording notes and recipes.
- Get ready to investigate the fascinating realm of fertility recipe cooking with a curious and open mind.
- Recall that the goal of this trip is to support your body and spirit as you pursue your

aspirations of being a mother and getting pregnant.

Now that you know the basics of cooking fertility recipes and the significance of diet for fertility, you're prepared to start this life-changing journey. We'll go into more detail about particular recipes and food plans that can help you achieve your reproductive objectives in the upcoming chapters. As you proactively work to optimize your reproductive health, get ready to nourish yourself from the inside out.

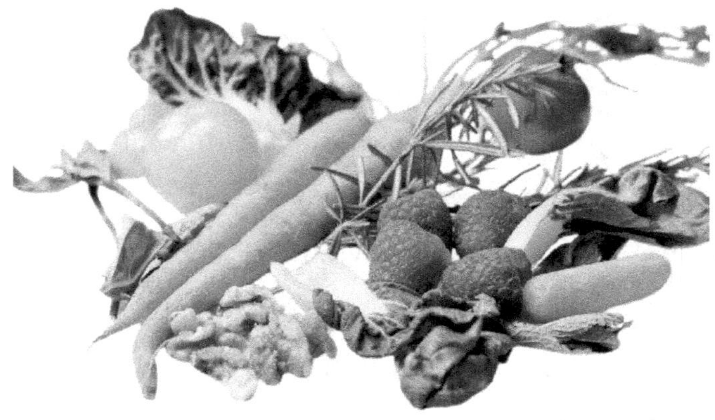

CHAPTER 2

Fertility-Required Ingredients

We'll look at the staples you should keep in your fridge and pantry to prepare fertility recipes in this chapter. These items, which range from nutritious grains and lean proteins to nutrient-dense fruits and vegetables, will serve as the cornerstone of your fertility-friendly meals. Let's start by defining and comprehending the essential elements of a kitchen designed to increase fertility.

Whole Grains:

Whole grains are high in fiber, vitamins, and minerals. Examples of such grains are quinoa, brown rice, oats, and barley. For hormonal balance and reproductive health, these grains sustain steady blood sugar levels and offer long-lasting energy.

- Keep a range of healthy grains in your cupboard to use as the foundation for salads, soups, grain bowls, and breakfast items.

Colorful Vegetables and Leafy Greens

Fertility depends on the abundance of folate, iron, and antioxidants found in leafy greens like spinach, kale, and Swiss chard.

- Vegetables with vibrant colors, including tomatoes, bell peppers, and carrots, are rich in vitamins, minerals, and phytonutrients that help with reproduction.
- To make sure you're getting a wide variety of nutrients, try to include a rainbow of vegetables in your meals.

Lean Proteins

Amino acids, the building blocks of hormones and reproductive cells, are found in lean proteins, including fish, chicken, tofu, tempeh, and legumes.

- To reduce your exposure to hormones and pesticides, if possible, choose high-quality, organic sources of protein.
- To promote hormone production, overall fertility, and the health of your muscles, include a dish of protein in each meal.

Healthy Fats

Hormone production and reproductive function depend on the healthy fats found in avocados, nuts, seeds, and olive oil.

- In particular, omega-3 fatty acids are essential for controlling inflammation and preserving the quality of eggs.
- To maximize fertility and support hormonal balance, include sources of healthy fats in your meals and snacks.

Superfoods that Boost Fertility

- You can include some of the superfoods that are known to increase fertility in your dishes.

- Berries: abundant in antioxidants; nuts and seeds: a good source of protein and healthy fats; fatty fish: salmon is strong in omega-3 fatty acids.

- To get the most out of these superfoods' benefits for fertility, try including them in your meals.

Herbs and Spices

Adding taste to your food is just one of the many health advantages of using herbs and spices.

- For instance, ginger may lessen inflammation and aid in digestion, while cinnamon might help control blood sugar levels.

- To improve the taste and nutritional value of your meals, experiment with different herbs and spices and have a well-stocked spice rack.

Vital Hydration

Water consumption is essential for both general health and fertility, so make sure you sip on plenty of it throughout the day.

- Herbal teas with added health advantages, such as those containing peppermint, chamomile, and raspberry leaf, can also be hydrating.
- Reduce your intake of sugary and caffeinated drinks because too much caffeine can harm your ability to conceive.

Having these staples in your kitchen will give you all you need to make scrumptious, healthful meals that help you achieve your fertility objectives. We'll employ these components in a range of fertility-boosting recipes tailored especially for women over 35 in the upcoming chapters. As you embark on your journey to enhanced fertility, get ready to fire your culinary creativity and nurture your body from the inside out.

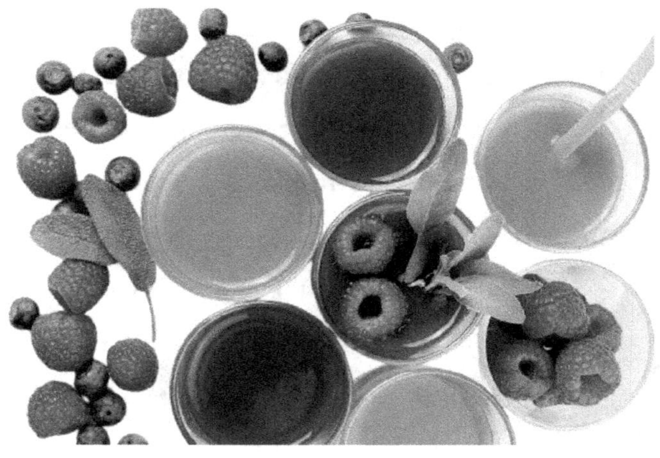

CHAPTER 3

Preparing Your Kitchen for Fertility Cooking

Within the scope of this chapter, we will concentrate on organizing and preparing your kitchen for the preparation of fertility cookbook recipes. Having a well-prepared kitchen will make the process of cooking more efficient and will make it simpler for you to incorporate items that are beneficial to fertility throughout your meals. Let's get into the stages of setting up your kitchen for success.

clear and clean your kitchen countertops

cabinets, and pantry to create a clean and organized workspace. To begin, you will need to clear the debris from these areas.

- The surfaces should be cleaned, the appliances should be cleaned, and any extraneous stuff should be decluttered to make room for your fertility-friendly ingredients and instruments.
- Not only will a clean and organized kitchen make your time spent in the kitchen more enjoyable, but it will also help you feel more at ease and more focused.

Taking inventory of your pantry staples and getting rid of any goods that have expired or are not being used is the second step in organizing your pantry.

It will be much simpler for you to find the things you need when you are cooking if you organize the shelves in your pantry according to categories such as grains, canned goods, spices, and condiments.

- If you want to keep your supplies fresh and conveniently accessible, you should think about investing in storage containers and labeling.

Putting Food in Your Refrigerator and Freezer

- Make space in your refrigerator and freezer for fresh veggies, lean proteins, and other perishable products.
- Keep fruits and vegetables visible and easily available to encourage frequent eating.
- Consider batch-cooking and freezing meals for busy days when you need a quick and nutritious option.

Important Kitchen Utensils and Equipment

- Gather important kitchen utensils and equipment for fertility recipe cooking, including: - Cutting boards and knives for slicing fruits, vegetables, and other components.
- Pots and pans of various sizes for cooking grains, meats, and veggies.
- Mixing bowls and tools for making and serving meals.
- Blender or food processor for preparing smoothies, sauces, and dressings.
- Measuring cups and spoons for correctly portioning ingredients.
- Having the correct tools on hand will make meal preparation more effective and pleasurable.

Creating a Meal Planning and Prepping Schedule

- Develop a meal planning and prepping regimen to streamline your cooking process and save time during hectic weekdays.
- Choose one day each week to plan your meals, develop a shopping list, and prep ingredients such as washing and slicing veggies.
- Consider batch-cooking fundamental ingredients like grains, beans, and meats to use in numerous meals throughout the week.
- By planning and prepping ahead, you'll ensure that you have nutritious meals ready to enjoy, even on hectic days.

Setting Up a Cooking Environment

- Create a comfortable and attractive cooking environment by adding personal touches such as music, aromatherapy, or natural light.

- Wear comfortable clothing and aprons to protect your clothes from spills and splatters while cooking.

- Invite family members or friends to join you in the kitchen to make cooking a communal and fun experience.

Practicing Kitchen Safety

- Prioritize kitchen safety by following proper food handling and storage standards.

- Wash hands well before and after handling food, and use separate cutting boards for raw meat, poultry, and produce to prevent cross-contamination.

- Cook items to the appropriate internal temperature and refrigerate leftovers promptly to prevent foodborne disease.

By following these steps, you'll establish a kitchen atmosphere that supports your fertility journey and makes it easier to incorporate nutritious meals into your daily routine. In the next chapters, we'll put your tidy kitchen and key tools to use as we dig into delectable fertility-boosting dishes for women over 35. Get ready to unleash your culinary imagination and nourish your body with meals meant to increase fertility and promote general well-being.

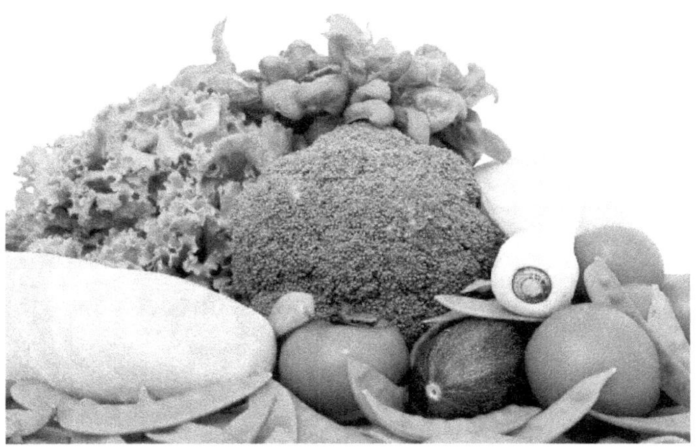

CHAPTER 4

Breakfasts for Fertility

In this chapter, we'll focus on producing tasty and healthy breakfasts customized to enhance fertility in women over 35. Starting your day with a balanced and nutrient-rich lunch sets the tone for optimum hormonal balance and reproductive health. Let's explore several fertility-boosting breakfast alternatives and give step-by-step directions for making them.

Fertility-Boosting Smoothies

- Choose a mix of fruits and vegetables rich in antioxidants, vitamins, and minerals to create a nutrient-packed smoothie.
- Combine items such as spinach, kale, berries, avocado, banana, and nuts or seeds

with a liquid base such as almond milk, coconut water, or yogurt.

- Blend until smooth and creamy, adjusting the consistency with extra liquid as required.

- Serve immediately or pour into a portable container for an on-the-go breakfast alternative.

Nutrient-Rich Oatmeal Bowls

- Start with a foundation of rolled oats cooked in water or milk of your choosing, such as almond milk or coconut milk.

- Add toppings such as sliced bananas, berries, chopped nuts or seeds, and a drizzle of honey or maple syrup for sweetness.

- Incorporate fertility-boosting foods like chia seeds, flaxseeds, and hemp seeds for increased protein, fiber, and omega-3 fatty acids.

- Customize your oatmeal dish to fit your taste preferences and nutritional needs.

Protein-Packed Egg Dishes

- Whip up a quick and easy egg meal such as scrambled eggs, omelets, or frittatas filled with veggies.

- Sautee veggies such as spinach, bell peppers, onions, and mushrooms until soft, then add beaten eggs and simmer until set.

- Season with herbs and spices like garlic powder, onion powder, paprika, and fresh herbs like parsley or chives.

- Serve alongside whole grain bread or avocado for a pleasant and nutritious breakfast.

Fertility-Focused Breakfast Bowls

- Create a breakfast bowl with a variety of grains, proteins, veggies, and healthy fats.

- Start with a foundation of vegetables, quinoa, brown rice, or farro, then top with lean protein such as grilled chicken, tofu, or beans.

- Add roasted or sautéed vegetables, such as sweet potatoes, Brussels sprouts, and broccoli, for extra nutrition and taste.
- Finish with a drizzle of olive oil, a sprinkling of seeds, and a dollop of Greek yogurt or avocado for richness.

Overnight Oats for Convenience

- Prepare overnight oats by mixing rolled oats with your choice of milk, yogurt, or plant-based substitute in a jar or container.
- Add flavorings such as vanilla essence, cinnamon, or cocoa powder, then sweeten with honey, maple syrup, or mashed banana.
- Stir in toppings like chopped nuts, dried fruit, and seeds, then chill overnight to let the oats soften and flavors mingle.
- Enjoy cold or warm the next morning, adding additional toppings as desired.

Balancing Macronutrients for Fertility

- Aim to incorporate a balance of carbs, proteins, and fats in your breakfast to give continuous energy and promote hormone synthesis.

- Incorporate whole grains, lean meats, and healthy fats into your morning meals to enhance satiety and regulate blood sugar levels.

- Experiment with different mixes and flavors to make your breakfasts new and pleasurable.

By including these fertility-boosting breakfast alternatives in your daily routine, you'll fuel your body with critical nutrients and enhance reproductive health. Experiment with different recipes and ingredients to find what works best for you, and enjoy the advantages of starting your day on a nutritious and tasty note. In the next chapters,

We'll explore fertility recipe cooking with lunch, supper, snacks, and beverages geared exclusively for women over 35.

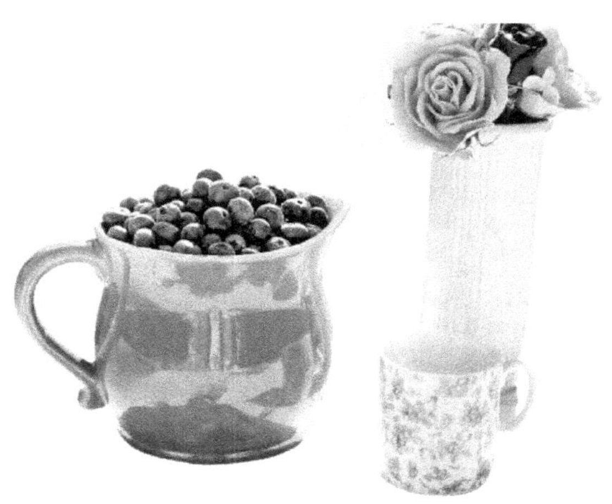

CHAPTER 5

Lunches for Fertility

In this chapter, we'll look at how to make healthy and nutritious lunches for women over 35 to help them conceive. A well-balanced midday meal gives you the energy and nutrition you need to get through the day while also encouraging good reproductive health. Let's look at a selection of fertility-boosting lunch alternatives and give step-by-step directions for making them.

Colorful Salad Creations

- For a nutrient-dense foundation, start with leafy greens like spinach, kale, or mixed greens.

- Include a range of bright veggies, such as bell peppers, cucumbers, cherry tomatoes, and shredded carrots, to boost vitamins, minerals, and antioxidants.

- Lean proteins like grilled chicken, tofu, chickpeas, and hard-boiled eggs can help with muscle function and hormone synthesis.

- To add fullness and taste, finish with healthy fats such as avocado slices, almonds, seeds, or a drizzle of olive oil.

Create a satisfying grain bowl

By starting with cooked healthy grains like quinoa, brown rice, or farro.

- Top with roasted or sautéed veggies like sweet potatoes, Brussels sprouts, zucchini, and mushrooms for extra fiber and taste.

- Add a plant-based protein source, such as black beans, lentils, or edamame, to help with muscle health and hormone balance.

- Drizzle with a tasty dressing made from olive oil, lemon juice, balsamic vinegar, and herbs for a flavor boost.

Create a nutritious soup

With veggies, lentils, and whole grains for a delicious supper.

- Begin by sautéing aromatics like onion, garlic, and ginger in olive oil until fragrant.
- Add diced veggies, cooked beans or lentils, broth or water, and herbs and spices to taste.
- Simmer until the veggies are soft and the flavors have combined, then serve hot with a side of whole-grain bread or crackers.

Protein-rich wraps and Sandwiches

- Choose whole grain wraps or bread as the foundation for your sandwich or wrap to deliver fiber and long-lasting energy.

- Layer on lean protein sources like turkey, chicken, tuna, or hummus for muscular support and satiety.

- Add a variety of vegetables, such as lettuce, tomato, cucumber, and sprouts, to boost vitamins, minerals, and crunch.

- Finish with a creamy and flavorful avocado, mustard, or Greek yogurt-based dressing.

Balanced Buddha Bowls

Combine nutrient-dense items to create a visually pleasing and enjoyable meal.

- Begin with cooked grains or leafy greens, then add a mix of colorful veggies, proteins, and healthy fats.

- Add fertility-boosting nutrients like avocado, almonds, seeds, and legumes for extra nutrition and taste.

- Drizzle with a homemade or store-bought dressing to bring all of the tastes together, and have a balanced and nutritious meal.

Practice Mindful Eating and Meal Control

Pay attention to your hunger and fullness cues to control your meal sizes.

- Try to fill half of your plate with veggies, one-quarter with lean protein, and one-quarter with healthy grains or starchy vegetables.
- To avoid overeating and promote digestion, eat deliberately, savoring each bite, and stop when you're pleasantly full.

Incorporating these fertility-boosting lunch alternatives into your meal rotation will provide your body with the necessary nutrients while also supporting reproductive health. Experiment with different food and taste combinations to keep your meals interesting and tasty. In the coming chapters, we'll look at fertility recipe cooking with meals, snacks, and beverages designed exclusively for women over 35.

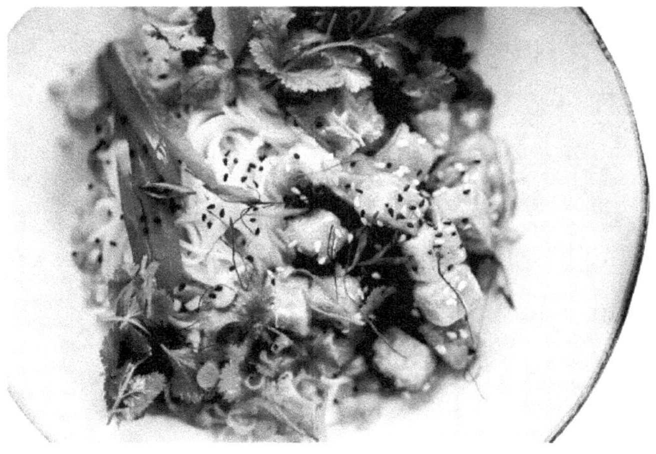

CHAPTER 6

Dinners for Fertility

In this chapter, we'll look at a selection of substantial and healthy supper recipes aimed at boosting fertility in women over 35. Dinner is an opportunity to recharge after a long day while providing your body with critical nutrients that promote reproductive health. Let's look at some fertility-boosting supper ideas and give step-by-step directions for making them.

One-Pot Meals for Easy Cleanup.

One-pot dinners are a quick and easy way to make a nutritious meal with little cleanup.

Choose robust soups, stews, or casseroles made with veggies, meats, and grains.

Begin by sautéing aromatics such as onions, garlic, and spices in a big saucepan or skillet.

Simmer veggies, proteins, grains, and liquids like

broth or coconut milk until everything is cooked and the tastes have blended.

Serve hot and enjoy a substantial and fulfilling supper that requires little work and cleanup.

Quickly cook flavorful stir-fries.

Stir-fries are a flexible and adjustable supper option that may be ready in minutes.

Begin by slicing your desired protein, such as chicken, tofu, or shrimp, into bite-sized pieces.

In a large pan or wok, heat the oil over medium-high heat. Add the protein, and cook until browned and cooked through.

Add veggies like bell peppers, broccoli, snap peas, and carrots, as well as garlic, ginger, and soy sauce, to taste.

Cook until the veggies are tender-crisp, then serve hot over prepared rice or noodles for a filling and healthy meal.

Step 3: Protein-Rich Main Dishes.

Choose protein-rich main courses like grilled salmon, roasted chicken, or lentil curry to help with muscle health and hormone production.

Marinate the protein in a delicious sauce or spice blend to enhance its taste and softness.

Grill, bake, or sauté protein until done, then serve hot with roasted or steamed veggies and nutritious grains for a complete meal.

Vegetarian and Plant-Based Options.

To enhance your fiber and plant-based protein intake, try vegetarian and plant-based meal alternatives such as blended vegetable stir-fries, tofu scrambles, and bean chili.

Try different varieties of beans and legumes, such as black beans, chickpeas, and lentils, to add texture and flavor to your dishes.

Use a variety of colorful veggies, herbs, and spices

to boost the flavor and nutritional content of your vegetarian recipes.

Balancing Macronutrients for Satisfaction

Aim for a combination of carbs, proteins, and healthy fats in your meal to give you long-lasting energy and promote hormone synthesis.

Include whole grains, lean meats, and healthy fats like avocado, almonds, and seeds in your dinners.

Experiment with different mixes and tastes to create pleasant and fulfilling dinners that help you achieve your reproductive objectives.

Enjoy Dinner Mindfully

Take time to chew each bite and appreciate the flavors and textures.

Eat carefully and listen to your hunger and fullness cues to avoid overeating and improve digestion.

Engage in discussion with family or loved ones to

create a comfortable and pleasurable meal environment.

By integrating these fertility-boosting supper alternatives into your meal plan, you will provide your body with the necessary nutrients while also supporting reproductive health. Experiment with different recipes and ingredients to keep your dinners interesting and fun. In the next chapters, we will continue to look at fertility recipe cooking with snacks, sweets, and beverages designed exclusively for women over 35.

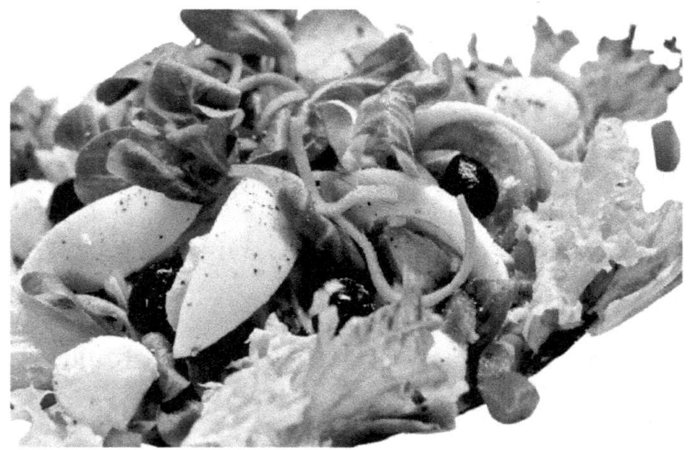

CHAPTER 7

Snacks and Desserts for Fertility

This chapter will look at tasty and enjoyable snack and dessert alternatives for women over 35 who want to be more fertile. Snacks may be a good source of nutrients and energy in between meals, but desserts can be enjoyed in moderation as a treat while still contributing to your overall fertility-focused diet. Let's look at a selection of fertility-boosting snack and dessert options and give step-by-step directions for making them.

Prepare energy-boosting snack balls.

Begin by adding rolled oats, nut butter (such as almond or peanut butter), and a natural sweetener like honey or maple syrup in a bowl.

- For added taste and texture, mix with chia seeds, flaxseeds, shredded coconut, and dried fruits.

- Mix until fully blended, then roll into bite-sized balls with your hands.

- Refrigerate the energy balls until hard, then serve as a quick and nutritious snack to fuel your day.

Prepare fruit-based treats

By slicing apples, bananas, strawberries, or kiwi into bite-size pieces.

- Dip the fruit slices in Greek yogurt or melted dark chocolate for extra taste and nutrition.

- Place the coated fruit slices on a baking sheet lined with parchment paper, then freeze until hard. Serve as a refreshing and delightful snack or dessert.

Healthy baked goods.

Make handmade baked products using nutritious ingredients, including whole grains, nuts, seeds, and natural sugars.

- Experiment with muffin, cookie, and bread recipes that contain fertility-boosting foods such as pumpkin puree, oats, walnuts, and dates.
- Enjoy these nutritious baked treats as a healthy snack or dessert that will satisfy your sweet tooth while helping you achieve your reproductive goals.

Create a nutritious and tasty yogurt parfait

layering Greek yogurt, fresh or frozen berries, granola, and nuts or seeds in a glass or dish.

- For more taste and sweetness, try adding honey, maple syrup, cinnamon, or shredded coconut to your parfait.

- Yogurt parfaits have a creamy texture and a pleasant taste, making them a simple snack or dessert option to assist your fertility journey.

Create a thick and creamy smoothie bowl

By combining fruits, veggies, Greek yogurt, and a drink of choice.

- Pour the smoothie into a bowl and garnish with granola, sliced fruit, almonds, seeds, and shredded coconut.
- Enjoy your smoothie bowl with a spoon, enjoying each bite and appreciating the flavors and textures of the ingredients.

Practice portion control and mindful eating to avoid overeating and increase satisfaction.

- Pay attention to your hunger and fullness cues, and stop eating when you are completely content.
- Select nutrient-dense snacks and sweets that provide a balanced macronutrient profile and complement your overall fertility-focused diet.

Incorporating these fertility-boosting snacks and desserts into your daily routine will provide your body with important nutrients while also supporting reproductive health. Experiment with different recipes and ingredients to discover your favorites, and get the advantages of eating tasty and nutritious snacks and sweets while on your fertility journey. In the next chapters, we will continue to look at fertility recipe cooking with beverages designed exclusively for women over 35.

CHAPTER 8

Fertility-Boosting Drinks

This chapter will cover a range of hydrating and fertility-enhancing drinks that are intended to assist women over 35 with their reproductive health. Fertility and general health depend on being hydrated, and certain drinks can boost reproductive health by adding extra nutrients and antioxidants. Now let's explore some fertility-friendly drink recipes and offer detailed preparation directions.

Fertility-Boosting Herbal Teas:

- Pick teas made from herbs like peppermint, chamomile, raspberry leaf, and nettle leaf that are proven to increase fertility.

- After 5 to 10 minutes of steeping a tea bag or loose tea leaves in hot water, filter and drink. Herbal teas are hydrating and full of healthy minerals and antioxidants that promote reproductive health. They may be sipped hot or cold.

Smoothies High in Nutrients

- Blend a range of fruits, veggies, and fertility-enhancing components to create nutrient-dense smoothies.
- For sweetness and taste, add fruits like berries, bananas, and mango after starting with a liquid base like almond milk, coconut water, or herbal tea.
- For extra nutrition and fullness, include leafy greens like spinach or kale and protein sources like tofu, Greek yogurt, or protein powder.

- Blend until creamy and smooth. Transfer to a glass and serve as a reviving and filling drink.

Infused Waters

- To make infused water, cut up fruits, vegetables, and herbs, then pour the mixture into a pitcher and let it steep for a few hours or overnight.
- For tasty and refreshing infused waters, use ingredients like cucumber, lemon, lime, berries, mint, and basil.
- Serve cold over ice as a rejuvenating and hydrating drink that promotes general health and fertility.

Green Juices

- For a nutrient-rich drink, blend leafy greens, fruits, and vegetables to make green juices.

- Juice such vegetables as spinach, kale, celery, cucumber, apple, and lemon using a juicer.

- For a simple and quick approach to increasing your intake of vitamins, minerals, and antioxidants, pour the green juice into a glass and drink it right away.

Alternatives to Dairy-Free Milk

- For a wholesome and lactose-free choice, go for dairy-free milk substitutes like almond, coconut, or oat milk.

- To support your fertility-focused diet, use dairy-free milk in place of cow's milk in smoothies, cereal, coffee, or tea.

- Seek out fortified dairy-free milk options that offer extra minerals for general health and reproductive assistance, such as calcium, vitamin D, and B vitamins.

Reducing Alcohol and Caffeine

- Reducing alcohol and caffeine intake can have a detrimental effect on fertility. Examples of these beverages include energy drinks, tea, and coffee.
- Go for decaffeinated versions of your favorite drinks or, as an alternative, caffeine-free herbal teas.

Reduce your alcohol intake since it can mess with hormone balance and reproductive health. Try reducing your use of alcohol to special occasions and, wherever you can, choosing mocktails or non-alcoholic beverages instead of alcoholic ones.

You may maintain your reproductive health, increase your chances of conception, and keep hydrated by making these fertility-boosting drinks a part of your routine. Enjoy the advantages of being hydrated and fed during your fertility journey by experimenting with different tastes and combinations to see which ones you like most. We'll continue our discussion of preparing fertility-friendly recipes in the upcoming chapters, complete with meal plans and shopping lists designed especially for women over 35.

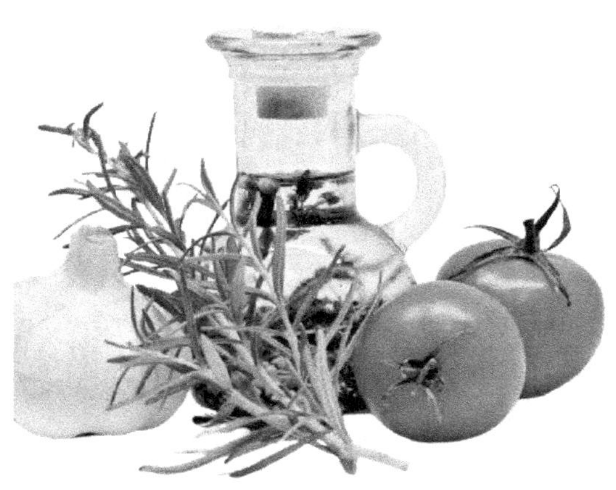

CHAPTER 9

A Fertility-Friendly Guide to Meal Planning and Shopping

In this chapter, we'll explore the significance of meal planning and offer a thorough how-to manual to help you organize your grocery shopping for preparing fertility recipes. Making a plan and preparing your kitchen with fertility-enhancing products will ensure that you are ready to cook scrumptious and healthful meals that promote reproductive health. Let's examine how to plan meals well and offer helpful advice for grocery shopping that works.

Recognizing the Advantages of Meal Planning

Meal planning is selecting the meals to be cooked throughout the next week and making a shopping list with the necessary items.

- Meal planning helps you save money and time, minimize food waste, and make sure you always have wholesome meals on hand.

- You can stick to your fertility-focused diet, choose healthier foods, and minimize stress and hurried decision-making by organizing your meals in advance.

Evaluating Your Dietary Preferences and Schedule

- When organizing your meals, take into account your weekly calendar, which includes social gatherings, family activities, and work obligations.

- Consider any nutritional requirements, food preferences, or dietary allergies that you or your family members may have.
- To keep your meals interesting and fulfilling throughout the week, try to strike a balance between flavors, textures, and nutrients.

Making a Meal Plan and Selecting Recipes

- Choose from a range of fertility-enhancing meals that suit your nutritional objectives and dietary preferences.
- Opt for recipes that are easily customizable and adaptable to changing seasons and ingredient preferences.
- Make a weekly meal plan that includes breakfasts, lunches, dinners, snacks, and drinks. Make a list of the recipes and supplies that you'll need for each meal.

Making a Shopping List

- Make a list of all the ingredients you'll need for the meals this week based on your meal plan.
- To make grocery shopping easier, group items on your shopping list according to categories like fruit, grains, proteins, dairy, and pantry essentials.
- To prevent buying duplicates, see whether there are any items in your cupboard or refrigerator. If so, mark them off your shopping list.

Tips for Grocery Shopping

- To reduce stress and save time, schedule your grocery shopping around a time when the store is less congested.
- Keep your attention on the supplies you'll need for your scheduled meals to help you

stick to your shopping list and resist impulsive buys.

- Save money on supplies and necessities by taking advantage of coupons, deals, and discounts.
- To cut costs and minimize food waste, think about buying products in bulk or frozen fruits and vegetables.

Getting Ready for Meal Prep

- Schedule a weekly period for meal prep, where you may pre-wash, cut, and prepare products.
- Preparing core foods like grains, meats, and sauces in bulk will help you save time and simplify meal preparation throughout the week.
- Until they are ready to use, store prepared items in airtight containers in the freezer or

refrigerator. Label them with the contents and date for simple identification.

These meal planning and grocery shopping processes will provide you with the tools you need to prepare scrumptious and nourishing meals that will help you reach your reproductive objectives. To maximize your chances of conception, plan and keep your kitchen stocked with fertility-boosting items to help you remain on track with your diet. We'll wrap off our exploration of the Fertility Recipe Cookbook for Women Over 35 with a recap of the most important lessons learned and parting reflections in the upcoming chapter.

CHAPTER 10

Summary and Main Points

Greetings on successfully finishing the Fertility Recipe Cookbook for Women Over 35! We've looked at a range of delectable and healthy dishes in this book that are designed to help women over 35 maintain and improve their fertility. Every food, from satiating snacks and sweets to filling dinners and nutrient-rich breakfasts, was thoughtfully created to include the vital nutrients and antioxidants required to maximize fertility.

When contemplating your fertility recipe cooking experience, keep the following points in mind:

1. Nutrient-Dense Diet: The vital nutrients and antioxidants required to promote reproductive health and improve fertility are found in a diet high in fruits, vegetables, whole grains, lean meats, and healthy fats.

2. Balanced Meals: To promote hormone synthesis and offer long-lasting energy, try to prepare meals that are balanced and contain a mix of carbs, proteins, and fats.

3. Meal Planning and Preparation: Keeping your fertility-focused diet on track and choosing healthier foods throughout the week depends on meal planning and preparation.

4. Hydration and Drinks: Make sure you stay well-hydrated by consuming lots of water and including fertility-enhancing drinks into your regular diet, such as smoothies, infused waters, and herbal teas.

5. Mindful Eating: Engage in mindful eating by focusing on your body's signals of hunger and fullness, appreciating every taste, and consuming meals without interruptions.

6. Community and Support: Be in the company of friends, family, and loved ones who appreciate and understand your infertility objectives. Joining online forums or support groups for women over 35 navigating the infertility process is something to think about.

Keep in mind that improving fertility with diet is a process that happens gradually and may require some time. As you progress toward better reproductive health, remember to set reasonable goals for yourself and acknowledge each accomplishment.

I urge you to try out various recipes, ingredients, and flavors as you proceed with your fertility journey to see what suits you the best. Make decisions based on your own needs and preferences by paying attention to your body and your instincts.

I appreciate you coming along on this gastronomic journey with me through the Fertility Recipe Cookbook for Women Over 35. I hope that these recipes will help you achieve your reproductive objectives, nurture your body, and provide you happiness and pleasure when you become a mother. I'm wishing you well, joy, and prosperity on your next adventure.

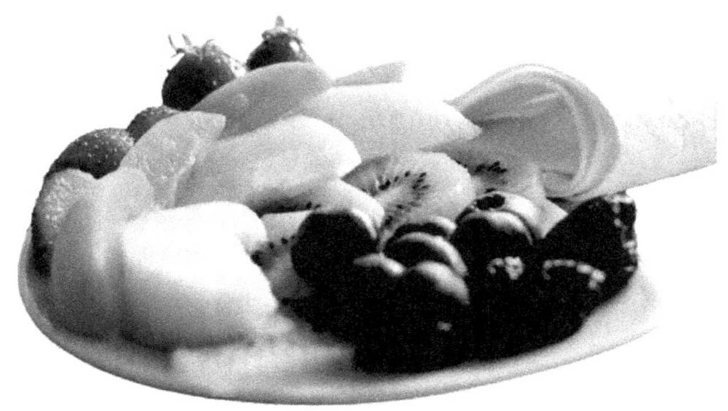

CONCLUSION

As we come to the end of our exploration of fertility foods, let us take a moment to consider the close relationship that exists between the wonder of life and food. Food has the transformational capacity to enhance reproductive health and kindle the spark of creativity. This has been discovered through the investigation of nutrient-rich ingredients, healthful recipes, and the joy of mindful eating.

However, our adventure is not over yet. With hope and wisdom at your disposal, may you keep appreciating the bountiful offerings of nature, relishing each mouthwatering morsel as evidence of the enduring power of the human body and the tenacity of the human spirit.

May you find comfort in knowing that you are surrounded by a community of spirits that share the goal of parenthood and are not alone on this journey. Let us unite in honoring the wonders of conception, the beauty of life, and the endless possibilities that lie ahead for those who dare to believe.

Thus, when you bid these pages farewell, may you take with you the knowledge acquired, the sustenance obtained, and the hope of fresh starts that each day brings. Because in the fertile garden, each seed sown is a murmured prayer, each meal shared is a blessing received, and each dream treasured is a journey accepted.

Meal Planner

Meal Planner

Month: _____ **Week:** ____

	Breakfast	Lunch	Dinner
Mon			
Tue			
Wed			
Thu			
Fri			
Sat			
Sun			

Grocery List

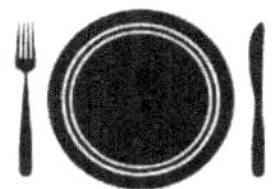

Meal Planner

Month: _______ **Week:**
____

	Breakfast	Lunch	Dinner

Mon

Tue

Wed

Thu

Fri

Sat

Sun

Grocery List

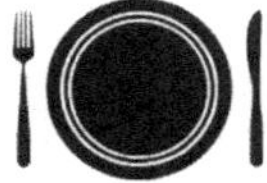

Meal Planner

Month: _____   Week: ___

	Breakfast	Lunch	Dinner
Mon			
Tue			
Wed			
Thu			
Fri			
Sat			
Sun			

Grocery List

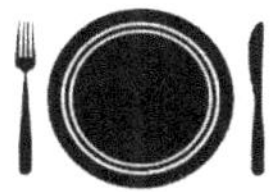

Meal Planner

Month: _____ **Week:** _____

	Breakfast	**Lunch**	**Dinner**
Mon			
Tue			
Wed			
Thu			
Fri			
Sat			
Sun			

Grocery List

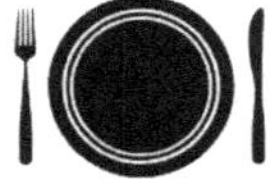

Meal Planner

Month: _____   **Week:** ___

	Breakfast	**Lunch**	**Dinner**
Mon			
Tue			
Wed			
Thu			
Fri			
Sat			
Sun			

Grocery List

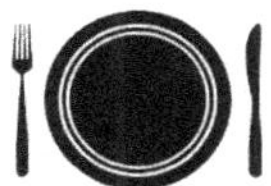

Meal Planner

Month: _____   **Week:**
_____

	Breakfast	**Lunch**	**Dinner**
Mon			
Tue			
Wed			
Thu			
Fri			
Sat			
Sun			

Grocery List

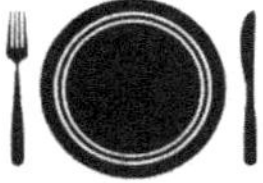

Meal Planner

Month: _____ **Week:** ___

	Breakfast	**Lunch**	**Dinner**
Mon			
Tue			
Wed			
Thu			
Fri			
Sat			
Sun			

Grocery List

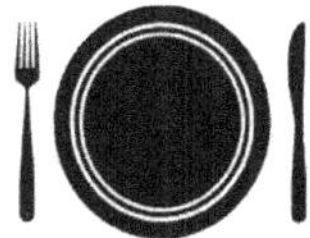

Meal Planner

Month: _____ **Week:** ___

	Breakfast	Lunch	Dinner
Mon			
Tue			
Wed			
Thu			
Fri			
Sat			
Sun			

Grocery List

Meal Planner

Month: _____ **Week:** _____

	Breakfast	Lunch	Dinner
Mon			
Tue			
Wed			
Thu			
Fri			
Sat			
Sun			

Grocery List

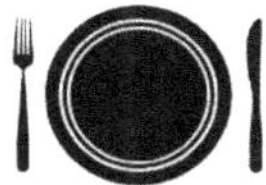

Meal Planner

Month: _____   **Week:** _____

	Breakfast	**Lunch**	**Dinner**
Mon			
Tue			
Wed			
Thu			
Fri			
Sat			
Sun			

Grocery List

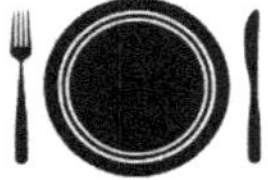

Meal Planner

Month: _____ **Week:**
_____

	Breakfast	**Lunch**	**Dinner**
Mon			
Tue			
Wed			
Thu			
Fri			
Sat			
Sun			

Grocery List

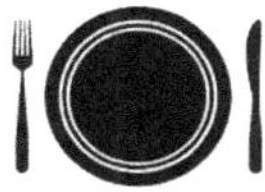

Meal Planner

Month: _____ **Week:** _____

	Breakfast	**Lunch**	**Dinner**
Mon			
Tue			
Wed			
Thu			
Fri			
Sat			
Sun			

Grocery List

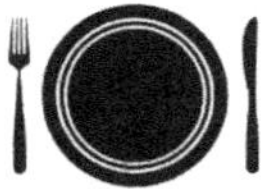

Meal Planner

Month: _____   **Week:** ___

	Breakfast	**Lunch**	**Dinner**
Mon			
Tue			
Wed			
Thu			
Fri			
Sat			
Sun			

Grocery List

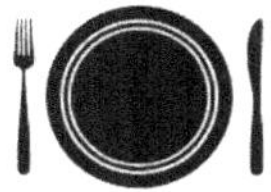

Meal Planner

Month: _____ **Week:** _____

	Breakfast	**Lunch**	**Dinner**
Mon			
Tue			
Wed			
Thu			
Fri			
Sat			
Sun			

Grocery List

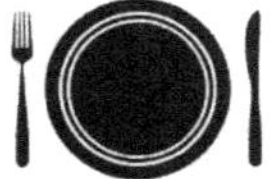

Meal Planner

Month: _____ **Week:** _____

	Breakfast	Lunch	Dinner
Mon			
Tue			
Wed			
Thu			
Fri			
Sat			
Sun			

Grocery List

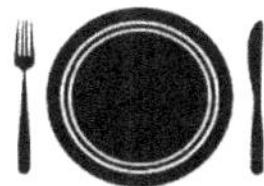

Meal Planner

Month: _____   **Week:** ___

	Breakfast	Lunch	Dinner
Mon			
Tue			
Wed			
Thu			
Fri			
Sat			
Sun			

Grocery List

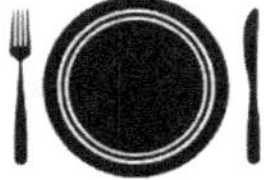

Meal Planner

Month: _____ **Week:** ____

	Breakfast	Lunch	Dinner
Mon			
Tue			
Wed			
Thu			
Fri			
Sat			
Sun			

Grocery List

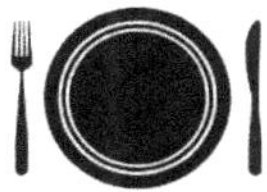

Meal Planner

Month: _____   **Week:** _____

	Breakfast	Lunch	Dinner
Mon			
Tue			
Wed			
Thu			
Fri			
Sat			
Sun			

Grocery List

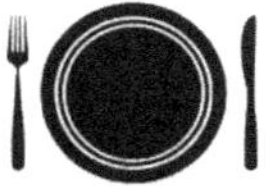

Meal Planner

Month: _____ **Week:** ___

	Breakfast	Lunch	Dinner
Mon			
Tue			
Wed			
Thu			
Fri			
Sat			
Sun			

Grocery List

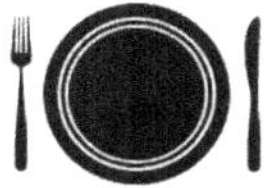

Meal Planner

Month: _____ **Week:** ___

	Breakfast	**Lunch**	**Dinner**
Mon			
Tue			
Wed			
Thu			
Fri			
Sat			
Sun			

Grocery List

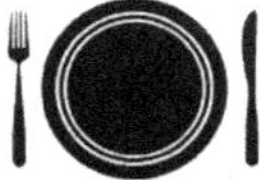

Meal Planner

Month: _____ **Week:** ___

	Breakfast	Lunch	Dinner
Mon			
Tue			
Wed			
Thu			
Fri			
Sat			
Sun			

Grocery List

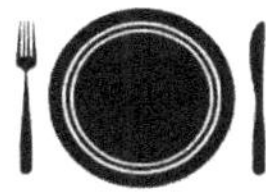

Meal Planner

Month: _____ **Week:** ____

	Breakfast	Lunch	Dinner
Mon			
Tue			
Wed			
Thu			
Fri			
Sat			
Sun			

Grocery List

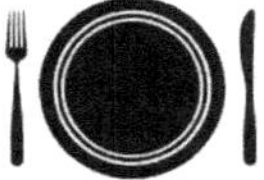

Meal Planner

Month: _____ **Week:** _____

	Breakfast	Lunch	Dinner
Mon			
Tue			
Wed			
Thu			
Fri			
Sat			
Sun			

Grocery List

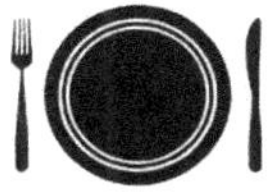

Meal Planner

Month: _____ **Week:**
_____

	Breakfast	Lunch	Dinner
Mon			
Tue			
Wed			
Thu			
Fri			
Sat			
Sun			

Grocery List

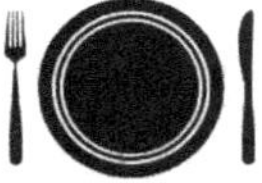

Meal Planner

Month: _______ **Week:** ___

	Breakfast	**Lunch**	**Dinner**
Mon			
Tue			
Wed			
Thu			
Fri			
Sat			
Sun			

Grocery List

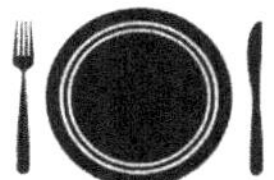

Meal Planner

Month: _____   Week:

_____

Breakfast   **Lunch**   **Dinner**

Mon

Tue

Wed

Thu

Fri

Sat

Sun

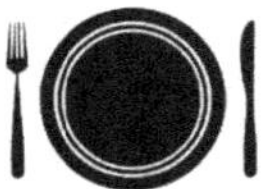

Meal Planner

Month: _____ **Week:** ____

	Breakfast	Lunch	Dinner
Mon			
Tue			
Wed			
Thu			
Fri			
Sat			
Sun			

Grocery List

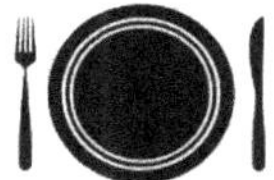

Meal Planner

Month: _____   Week:
____

	Breakfast	**Lunch**	**Dinner**
Mon			
Tue			
Wed			
Thu			
Fri			
Sat			
Sun			

Grocery List

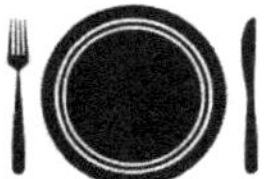

Meal Planner

Month: _____ **Week:** _____

	Breakfast	Lunch	Dinner
Mon			
Tue			
Wed			
Thu			
Fri			
Sat			
Sun			

Grocery List

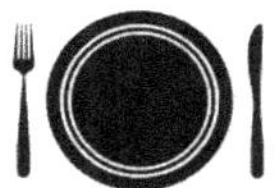

Meal Planner

Month: _____ **Week:** _____

	Breakfast	Lunch	Dinner
Mon			
Tue			
Wed			
Thu			
Fri			
Sat			
Sun			

Grocery List

Meal Planner

Month: _____ **Week:** ___

	Breakfast	Lunch	Dinner
Mon			
Tue			
Wed			
Thu			
Fri			
Sat			
Sun			

Grocery List

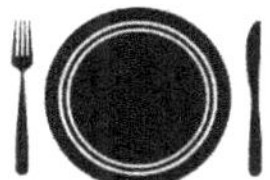

Meal Planner

Month: _____ **Week:** _____

	Breakfast	**Lunch**	**Dinner**
Mon			
Tue			
Wed			
Thu			
Fri			
Sat			
Sun			

Grocery List

Meal Planner

Month: _____ **Week:** _____

	Breakfast	Lunch	Dinner
Mon			
Tue			
Wed			
Thu			
Fri			
Sat			
Sun			

Grocery List

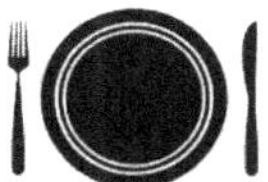

Meal Planner

Month: _____ **Week:** _____

	Breakfast	**Lunch**	**Dinner**
Mon			
Tue			
Wed			
Thu			
Fri			
Sat			
Sun			

Grocery List

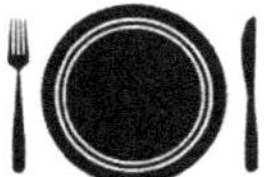

Meal Planner

Month: _____ **Week:**
_____

	Breakfast	Lunch	Dinner
Mon			
Tue			
Wed			
Thu			
Fri			
Sat			
Sun			

Grocery List

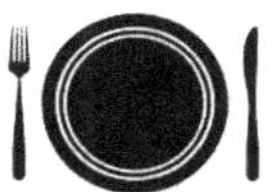

Meal Planner

Month: _____ **Week:** ___

	Breakfast	**Lunch**	**Dinner**
Mon			
Tue			
Wed			
Thu			
Fri			
Sat			
Sun			

Grocery List

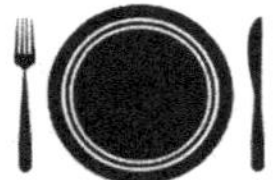

Meal Planner

Month: _____ **Week:** ___

	Breakfast	**Lunch**	**Dinner**
Mon			
Tue			
Wed			
Thu			
Fri			
Sat			
Sun			

Grocery List